W.T.H. IS IN YOUR FOOD?!

SUGAR-FREE IS NOT THE WAY TO BE!

TABLE OF CONTENTS

Thank you to all family and friends who believed in me. You all are truly amazing. I also want to give a special shout out to Eric Vaughn Black for his amazing support and consistent faith in me. I miss you my friend.

First and Foremost

This little book was written to merely introduce a personal opinion. It's based on my own independent research on the popular "low-calorie," "sugar-free," artificial sweeteners that have become a norm in today's food supply. I'm not a doctor or a scientist, and I haven't gone to school to be a certified nutritionist or dietician. I am just a normal (um, maybe a little weird) female who has a passion to keep our bodies clean and free of chemical containing foods.

From the beginning of time we were created to eat from the earth (fruits, nuts, etc.). Before men started meddling with our food supply everything was _natural_ and _organic_. There were no pesticides, chemicals sprayed in the atmosphere, synthetic fillers, and such. Everything was raw, natural, and pure. (The way it should be.) I do understand that these methods were meant to "increase our food supply," but trust me, there are more logical and less expensive ways to keep the bugs away! (For example: plant based oils, neem juice, cayenne pepper, etc.) I'm pretty sure I read or heard somewhere that we produce enough food to END WORLD hunger! With that being said, why are we still poisoning our food? #justwondering.

My sheer mission in life is to help lead others to the simplistic awareness, yet very relevant reality that chemicals, such as automotive antifreeze, (what?!) should not be used in our food supply and/or beverages. #forreal! (Yummy. Right!? Give it up for Propylene glycol!) That's it! That's my life's passion.

Learning little details about the smallest ingredient might seem trivial, but isn't our bodies all we really have? Health does matter for a good, focused, and better *feeling* life! We HAVE to start caring about the small details we are consuming in order to have full control of our overall health. A chemical here, or a toxin there, pretty soon we become a ticking time bomb. If you are feeling lethargic, apathetic, lacking physical and mental energy at all, spacey, or just plain blah, it may be what you are consuming on a daily basis.

Just think about it, when we scrape and cut open our skin, as long as we keep that wound *clean* and well-tended to, the body *easily* heals it. You don't even have to think about it. That is exactly how the interior of our anatomy works. Our bodies will **naturally** heal on their own if given the right nutrients. We have to eat clean to feel good and lively. If you keep your body clean from the inside out, it will do what it's meant to- keep you alive, energetic, focused, and consistently happy! When you *feel* good you are usually automatically in a good mood. Yes? or No? Good health= great life. Healthy living really does matter.

   *Please know and understand that anything written in this book is definitely not solid fact or truth – just a researched personal opinion. Certainly investigate it all yourself before you give credence to anything within.

Introduction: Empty Calories

It is said that millions of Americans now enjoy "low-calorie," "sugar-free" foods with enormous amounts of benefits to their overall health. Two well-known benefits being: weight loss and weight maintenance. Well, let's dig a little deeper and study these artificial sweeteners, as well as their potential side effects on our bodies.

Yo, I love sweet! You *probably,* (maybe, sort of) love sweet! We all scream for that sweet! Why? Well, it releases endorphines! Research has shown when you intake something sweet your brain releases dopamine. Dopamine is a *'feel good'* neurotransmitter. In other words, your brain's reward station. The hormone leptin is also released. Leptin sends an "I'm full" signal to your brain once you have consumed a sure amount of calories. Well, when you consume something sweet with **empty** calories dopamine is still activated, but the hormone leptin is *tricked.* There is nothing to fill you, so your body still *feels* hungry. Leptin is never deactivated because the calories were never there. Artificial sweeteners confuse your body because it thinks its receiving sugar which is normally accompanied with calories. It is deprived of the calories which causes your body to believe it needs *more*. (FEED ME!) Your body will then began to have carbohydrate cravings- (noooooo!) Those cravings are what potentially lead to that awful weight gain. Does that make sense?

So, if that is the case then why is it advertised that "sugar-free" which is typically "low-calorie" helps you lose weight? It definitely does. If you were drinking a sugary soda that contained 150 calories and then switched to a "sugar-free," "no-calorie" diet soda you will notice a change in your weight- at first. (uh?)

Okay, let me explain. I have two plausible reasons why "sugar-free" may be sabotaging your weight loss or weight maintenance. Let me bring in the professionals (lol).

1. There was a study where members in the San Antonio Heart Study drank more than 21 diet sodas a week. The study proved that they were twice as likely to become overweight or obese compared to the people who didn't drink diet soda. Why is this? Many studies have shown that sugar is addicting. If you are consuming something 200-2,000 times sweeter than natural sugar on daily basis your "sweet tooth" tolerance is sky high. It trains your taste buds to crave sweets. The intense sweetness overstimulates the sweet receptors. This may cause you to dislike the sweetness in nutritional foods- it doesn't compare to that sugariness that your brain and body have adapted to; therefore, you

crave, and then eventually consume more foods high in fat, sugar, salt, and cholesterol. (Ahhhhh!)

2. Calories are so important for good health and consistent energy. When you began to decrease calories, and start eating and drinking foods with *zero* calories your body thinks it is being starved. It goes into survival mode. This causes your body to hang on to every calorie you do consume. This is the exact opposite of what you want! Your body thrives on calories! If you are a calorie counter, figure out how many calories you need a day and eat *real* foods that contain calories. Eating a "sugar-free," "low-calorie" pack of cookies is just tricking your body and sabotaging your weight lose.

To conclude, if something is labeled "sugar-free" or "low-calorie" it does not necessarily mean it is *better*, *safer*, or *healthier* for you. You have to understand how your body processes the artificial ingredient, chemical, or sugar substitute.

14

Hmmm.. GMOs?

W.T.H. is GMO? Frankly, some of these artificial sweeteners have GMOs in them. For that reason, I'll go ahead and give a very short analogy of what genetically modified organisms (GMOs) are.

A GMO is simply an organism that has been genetically modified. Scientist wanted to make crops that were more resilient to external conditions (rain, snow, cold, heat, insect infestations, etc.). So, they discovered a way to take DNA from one organism and put it in another. For example: Take a crop of peppers. Let's say overnight the temperature went down to a freezing degree which caused the peppers to become frozen. They could no longer sell the peppers. In order to fix this, they obtained DNA from another organism that COULD withstand freezing temperatures and placed it in the peppers; such as, the DNA of an arctic fish. Arctic fish can withstand freezing temperatures; therefore, placing this in a crop of peppers will increase the chance of 100% crop yield without it freezing. And how do they get the DNA of an arctic fish into a peppers DNA? Well, in order to invade one cell with another organism's DNA you have to place a virus or bacteria within it for it to attach or invade that cell, otherwise the foreign cell will be *rejected*. This is where the problem of GMO food begins: viruses and bacteria's that are being implanted in the healthiest foods our green planet has to offer us.

I will not go any further with the details of GMOs simply because the main focal point for this book is artificial sweeteners. I would, however; urge you to research it on your own.

To quickly sum it up, the idea was to (once again) potentially assist with world hunger. How is injecting our fruits and vegetables with viruses and bacteria healthy or helping that situation? MMM...?

The List

First, let's start with a list of the "low-calorie," "sugar-free," artificial sweeteners. Some are similar in chemical compound and structure, but may have different calories per gram, glycemic index, effects, and flavor. This is just to get you acquainted with the names of the artificial sweeteners. I suggest reading over them twice-maybe three times. That way, if you decide to start reading the list of ingredients on a product, you will recognize them. And then eventually know if they are beneficial for your health, or the exact opposite.

Side Note: I have seen where a product will say "no aspartame," yet had

acesulfame potassium as the sweetener
which is just as harmful, and sometimes
even has aspartame mixed within it. (We
will get to all that later.) Please realize that
the *Also known as* is just as important! It
may seem like a lot at first, but trust me-like
with everything- it gets easier in time. Have
fun!

- **Acesulfame Potassium (E950)**
  Also known as:
  - ✧ Acesulfame K
  - ✧ Ace K
  - ✧ ACE

- **Advantame**

- **Alitame (E956)**

- **Aspartame (E951)**
  Also known as:
  - ✧ Acesulfame Potassium
  - ✧ APM

◇ Aspartyl-phenylalanine-1-methyl ester

- **Aspartame-acesulfame salt (E962)**

- **Cyclamate (E952)**
  Also known as:
  ◇ Calcium Cyclamate
  ◇ Cyclamic Acid
  ◇ Sodium cyclamate

- **Erythritol (E968)**
  Also known as:
  ◇ Erythrite
  ◇ Meso-erythritol
  ◇ Tetrahydroxy butane

- **Hydrogenated Starch Hydrolysates (HSH)**
  Also known as:
  ◇ Hydrogenated Glucose Syrup
  ◇ Maltitol Syrup
  ◇ Sorbitol Syrup

- **Isomalt (E953)**
  Also known as:
    ✧ Isomoltitol
    ✧ Hydrogenated Isomaltulose

- **Lactitol (E966)**
  Also known as:
    ✧ Lactit
    ✧ Lactobiosit
    ✧ Lactositol

- **Luo Han Guo Fruit Extracts**
  Also known as:
    ✧ Monk Fruit

- **Maltitol (E965)**
  Also Known as:
    ✧ D-Maltitol
    ✧ Dried Maltitol Syrup
    ✧ Hydrogenated Glucose Syrup
    ✧ Hydrogenated High
      Maltose-Content Glucose Syrup
    ✧ Hydrogenated Maltose
    ✧ Maltitol Syrup Powder

- **Mannitol (E421)**
  Also known as:
  - Mannite
  - D-Mannitol

- **Neohesperidin dihydrochalcone (E959)**
  Also known as:
  - Neohesperidin DC or NHDC

- **Neotame (E961)**

- **Saccharin (E954)**
  Also known as:
  - Sodium saccharin
  - Calcium saccharin
  - Acid saccharin
  - Potassium saccharin

- **Sorbitol (E420)**
  Also known as:
  - D-Glucitol
  - D-Glucitol syrup
  - Sorbit

- ✧ D-Sorbitol
- ✧ Sorbol

- **Steviol Glycoside**
  Also known as:
  - ✧ Rebaudioside A
  - ✧ Rebaudioside C
  - ✧ Reb-A
  - ✧ Rebiana
  - ✧ Stevioside

- **Sucralose (E955)**
  Also known as:
  - ✧ 4,1,6'-trichlorogalactosurcrose

- **Tagatose**
  Also known as:
  - ✧ Naturlose®

- **Xylitol (E967)**

The Breakdown

Now I'd like to do a very brief breakdown of all the artificial sweeteners that I could find. I encourage you to do your own research and familiarize yourself with each one.

- **Acesulfame Potassium (E950)**
  Also known as:
    - Acesulfame K
    - Ace K
    - ACE
    - Sunett

Pros:

- ✓ 0 Calories per gram.
- ✓ Glycemic Index: 0.
- ✓ F.D.A Approved.
- ✓ Requires labeling.

✓ 90 studies support its safety.

Cons:

➢ Contains Methylene Chloride.
➢ OSHA 3144-06R 2003 considers it to be "potential occupational carcinogen."
➢ Used as a propellant, paint stripper, and degreaser.
➢ Long term exposure may cause:
- Mood swings/Mental confusion.
- Depression.
- Headaches.
- Nausea.
- Impaired eyesight.
- Potential cancer.
- Hypoglycemia.
- Damage to liver and kidneys.
- Affect thyroid which may

lead to weight gain.

Wait. Hold UP! This sweetener is also used as a propellant, paint stripper, and degreaser!? And they use it in our delicious food and drinks. #SaveUsAll! #lol

Acesulfame K is 200 times sweeter than table sugar (which means they can **use less to sweeten** the product). It is also used as a flavor enhancer or to preserve the sweetness in the food. It is found in soft drinks, candies, canned foods, baked goods etc. There has been quite a bit of opposition as to whether we should be using this synthetic chemical in our food supply, but the FDA is not requiring further testing. I personally would avoid this sweetener considering the potential negative side effects. Even *OSHA* considers it to be a carcinogen (cancer causing). If that's the case, why would we want to have this in our soft drinks, baked desserts, or even near us?

Brand names: Sunett®, Sweet One®, Swiss Sweet®, Sweet & Safe® (Sweet and *SAFE*...mmm… really? Safe you say?) (There may be more brands.)

- **Advantame**

Pros:

- ✓ 0 Calories per gram.
- ✓ Glycemic Index: 0.
- ✓ Approved by the FDA.
- ✓ Low Cost.
- ✓ Extend sweetness duration.
- ✓ Improve sweetness. (20,000 times sweeter than table sugar.)

Cons:

- ➢ Contains phenylalanine. (This is typically only harmful to those with phenylketonuria. Phenylketonuria is a rare disease– their bodies can't

metabolize phenylalanine.)
- ➢ Derived from Aspartame. (see aspartame)
- ➢ Contains Genetically Modified Organisms (GMOs).
- ➢ Doesn't require labeling.
- ➢ Manufacturing process is kept hidden.
- ➢ May Cause:
  - Headaches.
  - Nausea.
  - Dizziness.
  - Weakness.
  - Change in Heart Rate.
  - Breathing difficulty.
  - Insomnia.
  - Seizures.
  - Neurological reactions.

Advantame can be found in syrups, gelatins, jams, jellies, puddings, chewing gum, frostings, some sodas, etc.

There was a study done with mice on the safety of this artificial sweetener. By the conclusion of the study the ratio of mice that survived to the ones that died was below FDA's own scientific recommendations. Yet this artificial sweetener is used in our food supply. The FDA also does not require this to be labeled. (scary?) The reason is because the sweetness of these chemicals are so intense that they do not have to use as much in the product: therefore; it is less likely to approach toxic levels. #mmm?

Just to add a little piece of somewhat interesting information: the same company that produces most of the world's MSG and a supplier of aspartame makes this *wonderful* sweetener: Advantame.

It's derived from aspartame (page 33). Just like aspartame it doesn't contain **any** natural ingredients. The cons outweigh the pros. It's also known to irritate the thyroid which may promote weight gain. Are we not trying to do the opposite when we choose the "low-calorie" and "sugar-free" options?

Since this is one of the newer artificial sweeteners there is not yet any brand names associated with Advantame.

- **Alitame: (E956)**

Pros:

- ✓ 0 calories per gram.
- ✓ Glycemic Index: 0.
- ✓ No aftertaste.
- ✓ 2,000 times sweeter. (They use such a small amount that it most likely will not cause harmful side effects.)
- ✓ Approved in the European

Union, Mexico, China, and
Australia.

Cons:

> Chemically similar to Aspartame.
> Not FDA approved in the United
  States.
> May still be used in the U.S. This
  isn't considered unlawful.
> No labeling required.

There isn't a lot of information that I
could find on Alitame. I would say due to
the similar chemical structure it has to
aspartame I personally would not consume.
It does NOT contain phenylalanine (refer to
Advantame), but it is formed from two
amino acids: aspartic acid and alanine.
These are 2 of the 3 ingredients in
aspartame. Aspartic acid is known as an
"excitatory" amino acid. It acts as a
passageway in the brain by assisting the

transmission of information from neuron to neuron. Too much aspartic acid in the brain kills certain neurons by allowing the influx of too much calcium. The reason it is called *"excitotoxin"* is because it excites the neural cells to **death** potentially causing chronic neurological disorders. (Is this why that first sip of a diet drink feels so good? Your neural cells get so *excited* that they keel over and die!) #SoIntense

Now, it is formed from amino acids that are found in the body so it may not contain GMOs. (yay!)
I mean, Does potential brain damage sound worth it to you though?

The brand name is Aclame®.

- **Aspartame (E951)**
  Also known as:
  - ✧ Acesulfame Potassium
  - ✧ APM
  - ✧ Aspartyl-phenylalanine-1-methyl

ester

Pros:

- ✓ 4 Calories per gram.
- ✓ FDA approved.
- ✓ Glycemic Index: 0.
- ✓ Requires labeling.
- ✓ Most researched food additive to date.
- ✓ 200 times sweeter than sugar.

Cons:

- ➤ Contains phenylalanine, Aspartic acid, and Methanol.
- ➤ Completely synthetic chemical combinations.
- ➤ **More adverse health conditions than all food additives *combined.***
- ➤ Non-Nutritive (**no nutritional

value).

➤ All brands or sweeteners with aspartame may contain GMOs.
➤ May Cause:
- Migraines/headaches.
- Stomach issues/abdominal cramps/pain.
- Heart palpitations.
- Vision impairment.
- High blood pressure.
- Insomnia.
- Memory loss.
- Dizziness.
- Hearing impairment.
- Birth defects.
- Hives/rash.
- Mood changes/depression.
- Joint pain.
- Diarrhea.
- Seizures and convulsions.

- Fatigue and weakness.
- Hallucinations.
- Increase cancer risk.
- Multiple Sclerosis (due to the methanol).
- Excitotoxicity (a phenomenon that occurs when cells receive excessive stimulation. They swell and then die- this can cause brain disease).
- May cause or contribute to Alzheimer's, or Parkinson.
- General dementia.
- Post-Polio syndrome.
- Epstein-Barr.
- Lyme disease.
- Graves' disease.
- Meniere's disease.
- ALS.

- Epilepsy.
- EMS.
- Hypothyroidism.
- Fibromyalgia.
- Lupus.
- Non-Hodgkin's.
- Lymphoma.
- Attention deficit disorder. (A.D.H.D.)

Oh my! Is this really still in the majority of our diet drinks and "sugar-free" foods? (EEEEKKKK!)

Aspartame changes once it enters the body. Here is what happens when you consume aspartame. Your body heat causes the aspartame to turn to wood alcohol. The wood alcohol then converts to formaldehyde (What? Gross!) and then to formic acid, (the sting found in fire ants) which in turn causes metabolic acidosis (this is when the kidneys are not removing enough acid from the body). The methanol toxicity acts like multiple sclerosis. Multiple sclerosis will not cause death, but methanol toxicity can.

If you are consuming a bottle or two of diet sodas, or possibly eating copious amounts of "sugar-free," "low-calorie" foods daily, or even regularly- you may want to reconsider if you are experiencing any of these side effects. The foods and beverages may contain aspartame. Honestly, It may be more beneficial to switch to foods and beverages made with natural sugar. Yes, natural sugars may have a slightly higher calorie content, but you may be saving yourself from laborious doctor visits. (Just sayin.) And HEY! If you keep reading you *will* find there are super healthy alternatives WITH zero calories that won't sabotage your weight goals! There is **always** an **alternative**. #KeepOnReading #IGotYou

There are other artificial sweeteners

that contain aspartame. In order to save on time, redundancy, and paper I will not reiterate the possible pros and cons of aspartame. Any artificial sweetener that does contain it has the same positive or negative side effects. *(There are quite a few.)*

Seriously though, this particular artificial sweetener irritates me. (I say that with love and genuine care.) For one, it's the most researched food additive to date! Second, it has more adverse health conditions then ALL food additives **COMBINED!** How in the world is this allowed to be in products we eat and buy daily?

Most candy, gum, sweets, diet treats, and drinks have aspartame or a sweetener that contains aspartame. Why? There are others that are proven better with *way less* side effects....

Brand names: NutraSweet®, Equal®,

Spoonful®, Sugar Twin® and
Equal-Measure®
(There may be more brands.)

- **Aspartame-acesulfame-salt (E962)**

Pros:

- ✓ 3 Calories.
- ✓ Approved by the FDA.
- ✓ Glycemic Index: 0.
- ✓ 350 times sweeter than table sugar.
- ✓ Approved for use in China, Russia, Hong-Kong, Australia, and New Zealand.
- ✓ All products are required to carry a **warning** label.

Cons:

- ➢ Contains **64%** *aspartame*.

➢ Contains 36% acesulfame potassium.
➢ Derived from GMOs.

Aspartame-acesulfame-salt is made by soaking a 2-1 mixture of aspartame and acesulfame potassium in an acidic solution and allowing it to crystallize- Bam! A sugar-like substance! Like I mentioned previously, if it contains aspartame than it potentially has the same side effects or benefits as aspartame. Since, it is 64% aspartame we can assume that it may be the same or similar.
Umm I'd say: "No eating this." #that's all.

▪ **Cyclamate (E952)**
Also known as:
✧ Calcium Cyclamate
✧ Cyclamic Acid

✧ Sodium cyclamate

Pros:
- ✓ 0 Calories per gram.
- ✓ Glycemic Index: 0.
- ✓ Used in over 100 countries.
- ✓ Oldest artificial sweetener.
- ✓ No GMO concerns.
- ✓ Pending re-approval by the FDA.
- ✓ Doesn't cause tooth decay.
- ✓ One of the cheapest sweeteners.
- ✓ Suitable for diabetics.
- ✓ May be labeled.

Cons:

- ➤ 30 times sweeter. That's 10% as sweet as other artificial sweeteners this means products may contain 10 times more in quantity.
- ➤ May irritate cancer.

➢ Doesn't occur naturally.
➢ Completely synthetic.
➢ Not currently FDA approved in the U.S.

This high intensity sweetener was used in the United States and then banned in 1970 for a potential connection to an increased risk in cancer, but is used in almost every other country. Cyclamate is found in tabletop sweeteners, soft drinks, instant beverages, dairy products, chocolate, chewing gum, candies, toothpaste, mouthwash, etc. It may be mixed with other artificial sweeteners: such as; saccharin, *aspartame*, sucralose, and acesulfame K to reduce the calorie content and enhance the sweet flavor. Most of these pros and cons speak for themselves. There isn't much need to expound. The main question I ask myself is: "If it is completely synthetic than why would I consume it?" It also is not approved by the

FDA, yet they may still use this in our food supply. This is not considered illegal.

Why is it that some products may have it listed others may not? Do they know that it irritates cancer and are trying to hide the fact that they use it?

(**Side note**: Sugars in general real or fake have been known to irritate cancer. Cyclamate (this sweetener) is used in a much larger quantity which could make it potentially more harmful.)

Brand names: Sucaryl®, Cologran® Assugrin®, Sweet'N Low®, and Sugar Twin®.

- **Erythritol (E968)**
  Also known as:
    ✦ Erythrite
    ✦ Meso-erythritol
    ✦ Tetrahydroxy butane

Pros:

✓ 0.2 Calories per gram.
✓ Glycemic Index: 0.
✓ FDA Approved.
✓ Occurs naturally in fruit.
✓ A sugar alcohol (meaning it has a small impact on blood sugar. It's helpful for those who are diabetic.)
✓ Doesn't promote tooth decay.
✓ Easy to digest.
✓ Non-carcinogenic.
✓ An antioxidant.
✓ Helps fight free radicals.
✓ Requires labeling.

Cons:

➢ May come from GMO corn.
➢ 70% as sweet as table sugar. It is not very sweet on its own, so it may be mixed other artificial sweeteners:

such as; aspartame, rebiana (from stevia), and sucralose.

➢ Too much can cause nausea.
➢ Expensive to produce.

This definitely sounds mostly safe. My only concern would be the genetically modified corn that it may be derived from. Other than that- I would trust it. I simply suggest getting the organic, non-GMO 100% **pure** erythritol if you were to purchase this. Or if it is mixed with another sweetener verify that the sweetener is plant based and pure as well. #BAM There you GO! A better sweetener. (There is more and even higher quality sweeteners to come.) #Exciting!

Brand names: ZSweet®, Wholesome Sweeteners®, Organic Zero®, Zerose®, Now Foods®, NuNaturals®, Swerve Natural Sweeteners®
(There may be more brands.)

- **Hydrogenated Starch Hydrolysates (HSH)**

  Also known as:
  ✧ Hydrogenated Glucose Syrup
  ✧ Maltitol Syrup
  ✧ Sorbitol Syrup

Pros:
  ✓ 3 Calories per gram.
  ✓ Glycemic Index: 36.
  ✓ FDA Approved.
  ✓ Approved in many other countries.
  ✓ Sugar alcohol (This means it has a small impact on blood sugar. It's helpful for those who are diabetic.)
  ✓ Doesn't promote tooth decay.
  ✓ Provides bulk and texture.

✓ Retains moisture.
✓ Helps keep appearance in foods products.
✓ Acts a preservative.
✓ Mask unpleasant flavors.
✓ May be labeled.

Cons:

➢ It's completely artificial (It does not occur naturally.)
➢ Usually made from modified corn starch (GMOs) or wheat (gluten).
➢ Lower sweetness than sugar.
➢ Mixed with other artificial sweeteners. (Acesulfame K, aspartame, neotame, saccharin, and sucralose.)
➢ May cause gastrointestinal discomfort in even small quantities.

➢ Has a laxative effect.

HSH is usually not sold on its own, it is mixed within other artificial sweeteners. It is also used in "sugar-free" candy and "low-calorie" foods. Hydrogenated Starch Hydrolysates seems to usually be used in conjunction with other sugar alcohols. If you recognize a sugar alcohol in an ingredient list or see *"sugar alcohol"* grams listed in the nutritional facts than it might have HSH within it. I would definitely look out for this on labels. You may have noticed in the *cons* that it may make you need to run to the bathroom more than you wish (laxative effect). Umm.. that doesn't sound pleasant. (lol)

- **Isomalt (E953)**
  Also known as:
  ✧ Isomoltitol
  ✧ Hydrogenated Isomaltulose

Pros:

- ✓ 2 calories.
- ✓ Glycemic index: 2.
- ✓ FDA Approved.
- ✓ Used in Australia, New Zealand, Canada, Mexico, Iran, and the European Union.
- ✓ A sugar alcohol. (This means it has a small impact on blood sugar. It's helpful for those who are diabetic.)
- ✓ Does not promote tooth decay.
- ✓ A nutritive sweetener. Derived from sugar beets.

Cons:

- ➤ May come from GMO beets.
- ➤ Too much may cause increased bowel movements, diarrhea, gas, and upset stomach. The body treats

it as a dietary fiber and may pass through the bowel in an undigested form.
- ➤ May be mixed with other artificial sweeteners to provide more sweetening power.
- ➤ Chemically manipulated.
- ➤ May be treated with acesulfame potassium to granulate it.
- ➤ Bad aftertaste.

My concern would be the the chemical manipulation, the fact that is may be mixed with other potentially harmful artificial sweeteners, and (of course) the potential GMO sugar beets. This artificial sweetener is typically used for a confectioner's sugar, but also can be found in candies, baked goods, chocolates, nutritional supplements, cough drops, etc.

Brand names: Decomalt®, DiabetiSweet®,

ClearCut®.
(There may be more brands.)

- **Lactitol (E966)**
  Also known as:
    ◇ Lactit
    ◇ Lactobiosit
    ◇ Lactositol

Pros:

  ✓ 2.4 Calories per gram.
  ✓ Glycemic Index: 0.
  ✓ Approved by the FDA.
  ✓ Approved in most countries.
  ✓ Sugar alcohol (It has a small impact on blood sugar- It's helpful for those who are diabetics.)
  ✓ Doesn't promote tooth decay.
  ✓ A nutritive sweetener (derived from nature: milk).

✓ Works as a prebiotic.
✓ In moderation it promotes colon health.
✓ No aftertaste.
✓ Good Flavor.

Cons:

➢ Derived from lactose or milk sugar. (Typically the cows are fed GMO grains).
➢ May cause diarrhea, gas, or cramping.

This sweetener seems perfectly safe unless you are lactose intolerant or have a dairy allergy. It can be found in ice cream, biscuits, chocolate, chewing gum, candies, etc. Just look for an organic, non-GMO product. The GMO grains that are fed to cows are not only harmful to them, but to us as well.

Brand names: LACTY®

- **Luo Han Guo Fruit** (*GREATness here!*)
  Also Known as:
  - ❖ **Monk Fruit**

Pros:

- ✓ 0 calories per gram.
- ✓ Glycemic Index: 0.
- ✓ Benefits known in China for 800+ years.
- ✓ 300 times as sweet as sugar.
- ✓ Contains important antioxidants.
- ✓ Good, clean taste.
- ✓ Supports the immune system, digestive tract, glands, and respiratory system.
- ✓ May help with allergies. (Calms the mast cells that release the chemicals

such as histamine- which is associated with allergies and asthma.)

- ✓ May help with Cancer.
- ✓ Fights Free Radicals.
- ✓ Acts as an anti-inflammatory.
- ✓ May have a powerful effect on diabetes.
- ✓ May assist with weight maintenance.
- ✓ May decrease risk of heart disease.
- ✓ Doesn't promote tooth decay.
- ✓ Considered one of the safest non-sugar sweeteners.
- ✓ Safe for those with Autism.
- ✓ No known concerns.
- ✓ Extracted naturally.

Cons:

- ➢ Some brands may contain

dextrose or other artificial
sweeteners, as well as GMOs.

Let me catch my breath... So, this
contains important antioxidants *and* it may
HELP with cancer?! What!? Well dang. This
seems pretty amazing! Like I said: "There is
always an alternative." I would definitely
just make sure you get the organic, **PURE**
goodness and you're all set!

For some reason there are brands
that take away the *saintly, pure* integrity of
Monk Fruit. They mix this amazing,
God-sent sweetener with dextrose and
other chemical/fake white, powdery
substances: a.k.a artificial sweeteners.
Please just watch out for those. #thanks.

Fun Facts: "Monk Fruit has been
used for centuries in eastern traditional
herbalism to increase chi and well-being,
earning the nickname: "**The Immortals
Fruit**."

~Back of Lakanto® sugar package.

Brand names: Purelo®, Virgin Extracts™, Lakanto®, Monk Fruit In The Raw®. *(In the Raw® I found to contain dextrose.)*

- **Maltitol (E965)**

  Also Known as:
  - ◇ D-Maltitol
  - ◇ Dried Maltitol Syrup
  - ◇ Hydrogenated Glucose Syrup
  - ◇ Hydrogenated High Maltose-Content Glucose Syrup
  - ◇ Hydrogenated Maltose
  - ◇ Maltitol Syrup Powder

<u>Pros</u>:

- ✓ 2 calories per gram.
- ✓ Glycemic Index: 36 for powdered. 52 for syrup.
- ✓ FDA Approved.

✓ A sugar alcohol. (It has a small impact on blood sugar- It's helpful for those who are diabetics.)
✓ Doesn't promote tooth decay.
✓ A nutritive sweetener. (Natural-Plant based.)

Cons:

➢ Derived from GMO corn syrup.
➢ Too much may cause bloating or gas.

The first thing I notice is the high glycemic index. This may cause you to have a high sugar rush and a fast crash. It seems pretty harmless compared to others. If you are purchasing this, or a product with this in it I would just look for certified organic, non-GMO brands.

Fun Fact: There were these little gummy bears that were an internet sensation for a bit. These little bears, and I quote caused: "volatile, poo-related escapades." This is all because of the lovely sweetener: *maltitol*. (LOL) SO! If you are constipated- eat up!

Brand names: Lesys®, Maltisweet®, SweetPearl®.

- **Mannitol (E421)**
  Also known as:
  - ✧ Mannite
  - ✧ D-Mannitol

Pros:

- ✓ 1.6 calories per gram.
- ✓ Glycemic Index: 0.
- ✓ Sugar alcohol (It has a small impact on blood sugar- It's helpful for those who are diabetics.)
- ✓ Doesn't promote tooth decay.
- ✓ A nutritive sweetener (derived from

nature: mushrooms, strawberries, onions etc.).

✓ Warning label required for laxative effect.

Cons:

➤ Synthesized from fructose which is derived from cornstarch. (Most corn starches are genetically modified.)

➤ Semi-artificially produced by adding hydrogen to fructose.

➤ Too much may cause diarrhea, stomach ache, or gas. (Mannitol attracts water from the intestinal wall called *osmotic effect.* This is what causes the diarrhea.)

This is a semi-artificially produced sweetener. I just don't like artificial. (yuck) There are other options that do not give a laxative effect or have these GMOs. (Why are they genetically engineering everything? Ahhh!)

- **Neohesperidin dihydrochalcone (E959)**
  Also known as:
  - ✧ Neohesperidin DC or NHDC

Pros:

- ✓ 0 calories per gram.
- ✓ Glycemic Index: 0.
- ✓ Approved in the European Union.
- ✓ Used to mask bitter flavors.
- ✓ May be labeled.

Cons:

- ➢ Not FDA approved.
- ➢ Chemically treated.
- ➢ May be combined with other

artificial sweeteners.

➢ Non-Nutritive (There is no nutritional value- it is not derived from nature.)

➢ May cause: nausea and migraines.

NHDC is more of a flavor enhancer than a sweetener. It is used for masking bitter flavors in food products, creates the creamy texture in dairy foods like ice cream and yogurt, reduces the bitterness in pharmaceutical drugs, used in condiments (ketchup and mayonnaise), and in animal feed, etc. It's completely synthetic and chemically created. #Healthy? For those reasons alone I would *maybe* try and steer clear if possible.

▪ **Neotame (E961)**

<u>Pros:</u>

✓ 0 calories per gram.
✓ Glycemic Index: 0.
✓ FDA approved.
✓ Approved in the European Union, Australia, and New Zealand.
✓ Most inexpensive Sweetener.
✓ No reported side effects due to the fact they use so little in each product. (7,000- 13,000 times sweeter than sugar.)
✓ Listed or labeled under the name E961.

Cons:

➢ Derived from aspartame.
➢ Non-nutritive sweetener. (Meaning it is not derived from nature.)
➢ Potential GMO ingredients.
➢ No labeling of "neotame" required

due to the small amount used.

This is mainly used by producers. It is sold as neotame, but isn't sold to the consumer market. It is chemically derived from aspartame which we now know is a known neurotoxin. It is found in chocolate, food supplements, pre-made salads, hard and soft candies, coffee and coffee substitutes, teas, dairy based desserts, water based flavored drinks, soups, etc. It may be labeled as "E961" on products. (Hopefully it's there.)

Saccharin (E954)

Also known as:
- Sodium saccharin
- Calcium saccharin
- Acid saccharin
- Potassium saccharin

Pros:

- ✓ 0 Calories per gram.
- ✓ FDA Approved.
- ✓ Glycemic Index: 0.

Cons:

- ➢ Mixed with other artificial sweeteners to mask metallic taste.
- ➢ Main ingredient is benzoic sulfimide.
- ➢ FDA classifies this as a "weak carcinogen."
- ➢ May contain GMOs because it is mixed with dextrose, which contains genetically modified organisms.
- ➢ No labeling required.
- ➢ May cause:
  - Allergic reactions for people who might have sulfa allergies.

- Diarrhea.
- Nausea.
- Skin problems or other allergy related symptoms.
- Cancer in bladder, ovaries, uterus, skin, blood vessels and other organs.

If it has the aforementioned side-effects and is considered a "weak carcinogen," than why would it not be labeled? Why is it used at all? (The FDA confuses me.) #Ha!

Brand Names: Sweet 'N Low®, Necta Sweet®, Cologran®, Hermesetas®, Sucaryl®, Sucron®, Sugar Twin®, Sweet 10®. (There may be more brands.)

- **Sorbitol (E420)**

Also known as:
- ✧ D-Glucitol
- ✧ D-Glucitol syrup
- ✧ Sorbit
- ✧ D-Sorbitol
- ✧ Sorbol

Pros:
- ✓ 2.6 calories per gram.
- ✓ Glycemic Index: 9.
- ✓ FDA approved.
- ✓ Occurs naturally in fruit.
- ✓ A cousin to natural sugar.
- ✓ Requires labeling to warn of laxative effect.

Cons:
- ➢ Made from glucose. (Glucose is derived from corn or corn starch- which is usually always genetically

modified.)

➢ Excessive amounts will cause diarrhea.

➢ Used as a medicine to relieve constipation.

➢ Mixed with other artificial sweeteners.

This seems safe(ish). You may now be familiar with my personal opinion. (lol) I would disagree with using sorbitol and why? GMO usage and the other artificial sweeteners that may be mixed within it. Let's not forget to mention that it's used as medicine to *relieve* constipation.(What the-EW.) It is sold as just *sorbitol* or within other artificial brands: therefore; there are not any brand names associated with this artificial sweetener, just Sorbitol.

- **Steviol Glycosides**
  Also known as:
  - ✧ Rebaudioside A
  - ✧ Rebaudioside C
  - ✧ Reb-A
  - ✧ Rebiana
  - ✧ Stevioside

Pros:

- ✓ 0 calories per gram.
- ✓ Glycemic Index: 0.
- ✓ FDA Approved.
- ✓ Approved in the European Union.
- ✓ Marketed as a "natural sweetener." (It is from stevia rebaudiana plant.)
- ✓ EFSA's reviews conclude that this is not carcinogenic or toxic.
- ✓ Does not pose a risk to pregnancy or children.

Cons:

> Mixed with other artificial sweeteners to mask bitter aftertaste (usually erythritol).
> May be mixed with dextrose- a corn derived sweetener. (Potential GMOs.)
> Numerous extraction methods. Some involve adding chloroform or hexane to the dry leaf.
> Calcium hydroxide and aluminum sulfate may be used to remove unwanted substances.
> No studies done for cancer risk.
> May cause:
  - Bloating.
  - Upset Stomach.
  - Gas.

- Allergies: itchy rash, mouth, or throat.
- Nausea.
- Vomiting.
- Diarrhea.
- Difficulty breathing.

This is safer than most. Most of the symptoms come from being allergic to the plant or the side effects from the artificial sweeteners it could be mixed with. Personally, I don't like the fact that we don't know if they used water, hexane, heat or any other chemicals to retrieve the stevioside. I've noticed a lot of the popular brands will say "natural or pure stevia," yet it is mixed with other artificial/chemical sweeteners (like dextrose). From what I've read, Stevia is usually highly processed with heat and chemicals that are not removed before selling. *(sad face)

Purchasing a pure, organic, non-GMO **liquid** form would probably be your best bet. You can also buy the plant, dry it out, steep it for 24 hours, and then strain the syrup for a homemade sweetener. I'm sure it's easy to grow. You can find the exact method online. It may be fun!

Brand names: Stevia®, Truvia®, Sweet Leaf®, NuStevia®, Stevia In The Raw®, and Now®: Better Stevia, Stevia Leaf Extract®.

- **Sucralose**
  Also known as:
  ♦ 4,1',6-trichlorogalactosucrose.
Pros:
  ✓ 3.3 Calories per gram.
  ✓ FDA Approved.

✓ Glycemic Index: 0.

✓ No effect on blood glucose.

✓ Doesn't promote tooth decay.

✓ May be labeled.

Cons:

➢ Contains dextrose and maltodextrin (which is usually derived from GMO corn).

➢ An organochlorine (A toxic substance used in *pesticides.*)

➢ Synthetic additives.

➢ Only 2 clinical studies were done before its approval. (36 humans total were studied in the trials).

➢ May cause or increase:

- Migraine.
- Stomach cramps.
- Muscle aches.
- Diarrhea.

- Bladder issues.
- Skin irritations.
- Inflammation.
- Dizziness.
- Shrinking of the thymus gland.
- Liver and kidney dysfunction.
- Reduces healthy intestinal bacteria.

Whew! Let me take a deep breath... Organochlorine? A **pesticide**? What? We're consuming something that is meant to *kill* pest? #OhMy

The story I recall reading is as follows: a scientist was making or tinkering with organochlorine, a chemical pesticide for cockroaches, rats, etc. As he was stirring and/or examining it- it splattered. A portion of the chemical landed on his face and he got a little taste of it. "OMG! this is sweet?! Let's take this cheap chemical and make bank off of it. Wait! Let's put it in a sunshine, yellow, bright package and call it Splenda® (what a splendid idea we have)."

Um. Do you think that we should be eating something that is used to kill bugs and small animals? What has this world come to? #Disturbing.

Disclaimer: The quotes are not based on any facts. Please research this all yourself. (Just having fun.)

Brand names: Splenda®, Nevella®.

- **Tagatose**
  Also Known as:
  - ✧ Naturlose®

Pros:
  - ✓ 1.5 calories per gram.
  - ✓ Glycemic Index: 0.
  - ✓ FDA Approved.
  - ✓ Approved in many countries.

✓ Great taste.
✓ Texture similar to sugar.
✓ Occurs naturally in small quantities in milk and some fruits, but doesn't contain lactose.
✓ Beneficial for diabetics.
✓ Doesn't promote tooth decay.
✓ A prebiotic.

Cons:

➢ Laxative effect.
➢ May cause: nausea or stomach cramps.
➢ It may be mixed with other artificial sweeteners.

Tagatose has not yet caught on as a sweetener so there is not much information on it. I'd say on its own it seems pretty harmless.

The only negative information that I

read is that it (like most all artificial sweeteners) is not absorbed by the body and is used only as energy. Other than that if you see this in a food product in the future- I wouldn't be too concerned, but always continue your research.

Brand names: PreSweet™Tagatose, AllSweet™Tagatose.

- **Xylitol (E967)**

Pros:

✓ 2 calories per gram.
✓ Glycemic Index: 7.
✓ Derived from nature. (Fruits and vegetables.)
✓ Resembles sugar in texture and taste.
✓ A sugar alcohol. (It has a small impact on blood sugar- It's helpful for those who are diabetics.)
✓ Doesn't promote tooth decay.

✓ 1-20 grams may reduce cavity formation.
✓ Using chewing gum with Xylitol may reduce bad bacteria in the mouth by 27-75%. (It doesn't affect the good bacteria.)
✓ Reduces the acidity of saliva.
✓ Increases absorption of calcium in the digestive system. (A prebiotic effect.)
✓ Daily use can reduce ear infections in children by 40%.

Cons:

➢ Almost always derived from corn which is almost always genetically modified.
➢ May cause
- Intestinal issues.
- Diarrhea.

- Gas.
- Bloating.

Xylitol is used in some toothpaste, chewing gums, mints, and other candies. To avoid the corn derived xylitol just look for an organic, non-GMO brand derived from birch trees. This sweetener seems harmless and actually may be good for you and your teeth. The chewing gum I purchase is sweetened with xylitol and its only $1.00! I definitely would prefer my toothpaste to be sweetened with this compared to what others use (**sodium saccharin, sucralose,** etc.). In fact, (I just checked) the toothpaste I use now is sweetened with "non-GMO xylitol." #sweet!

Brand names: Euphoria®, KAL®, Miracle Sweet®, Natures Provisions®, Now®, Perfect Sweet®, Poly Sweet®, Smart Sweet® (Organic Hardwood), Unique Sweet®, Vitamin Shoppe®, XyloPure®, XyloSweet® (There may be more brands.)

Other Sweeteners

There are so many different plants, chemicals, and methods to sweeten our food. Here are a few more that are not considered "sugar-free" or "low-calorie," but I feel are just as important to touch on.

Sucrose: (also called: saccharose)
- 16 calories per teaspoon.
- Common table sugar. (Consist of glucose and fructose.)
- Occurs naturally in fruit.
- Found in honey.
- Gives energy.
- A great preservative. (Slows the growth of bacteria and molds.)
- A chemical name for white sugar.
- Has no nutritional value.
- Excessive amounts have been linked to tooth decay, diabetes, and obesity.

This may seem a little confusing. How is it in fruit, but it may also cause diabetes or obesity? Is fruit not considered healthy? Consuming sucrose through fruit and honey, the natural sources, is completely safe. It's when they isolate it that it becomes unhealthy. Unfortunately, usually anytime any food product is isolated it is usually very processed and completely manipulates the chemical structure. This causes it to become unnatural, unhealthy and far from its original form.

Sucrose is very popular in the food industry. You may find this in many products. Just remember to read the ingredient list.

Glucose: (also called dextrose)
- Found in fruit and vegetables.
- Main fuel used by the body. (Vital to life.)
- Excellent in exercise and sport. (It

gives quick energy.)
- Very high glycemic index.
- Cheaper than cane sugar.
- Quickly raises blood sugar level.
- Harmful to teeth.
- A generic product. (Mostly sold as dextrose.)
- May contain GMOs.

Once again we should only consume this through its natural sources; such as: raw, organic, pure honey, or fruit. Any other form is unhealthy and has negative side effects.

Fructose:
- Small amounts found in fruit, honey, and vegetables.
- Low glycemic Index.
- Usually derived from corn (It may contain GMOs.)
- When consumed in high amounts it's turned immediately into fat.
- May cause:

o   Obesity.
o   Type 2 diabetes.
o   Heart Disease.
o   Gout.
o   Elevated blood pressure.
o   Fatty liver disease.
o   Insulin resistance.
o   Depletion of vitamins and
    minerals.
o   Increased appetite.
o   Arthritis.
o   Cancer.

On average, If you receive fructose from fruits and vegetables you'd intake about 15 grams a day. If you consume fructose through just sweetened beverages, than you are getting an average of 73 grams a day. It's not the fructose that is bad, but the amount we are consuming unnaturally. Fructose is not digested or produced by our bodies. When we consume too much fructose the liver goes into overload and turns it into fat. My opinion is to avoid this sweetener unless (once again) it comes from fruits or vegetables (preferably organic).

High Fructose Corn Syrup: (HFCS)
- 55% fructose and 42% glucose.
- Produced from corn starch. (May contain GMOs.)
- Half the price of sugar.
- Provides color in baked foods.
- Thickens and stabilizes processed food.
- Prolongs shelf life.
- Contains **mercury**.
- May cause:
  o Obesity.
  o Type 2 diabetes.
  o Heart Disease.
  o Elevated blood pressure.
  o Liver disease.
  o Increased appetite.
  o Cancer.
  o Irreversible brain and nervous system damage due

to high levels of mercury.

I'm sure we have all heard that High Fructose Corn Syrup is not the best to consume. This is very well-known now. Honestly, 5 minutes of research can prove this. Just look at the potential side effects: heart disease, cancer, obesity, diabetes, etc. There may also by toxic mercury in HFCS. There was study that tested HFCS and over 43% of the HFCS that was tested had high levels of mercury. Mercury has been known to cause neurological disorders. (Yet they still have this in our food?)

HFCS is still widely used in the food industry despite the known side effects and studies. It is found in everyday sodas, candies, breads, snacks, and the list can go on and on. Anytime I see this name I put the item right back. Thankfully, the awareness is increasing, We are now seeing a ton of other sweetener options. Even if it just says 'sugar' on the ingredient list (to me) that's better than 'High Fructose Corn Syrup.' I'd rather not risk irreversible brain damage. (Ya know what I mean?)

As we can all now certainly see we have *SO* many options when it comes to sweetening our food and beverages. There are many, many more sub-sweeteners that I did not go over. I just encourage you to research it all yourself and form your own opinion and lifestyle.

Sweet N' Simple

I'm sure you are all wondering, "How in the *WORLD* can I avoid all of this?" There *is* hope!

I will be straight-up and honest with you. Me personally, I **love** carbonated beverages, chocolate, candy, and anything sweet! I mean, who doesn't like something sweet every now and then?

The issue I have noticed with grabbing a quick sweet fix for myself at a local grocery store whether it be soda, candy, or chocolate is that the main sweetener in our food supply currently is that *lovely* High Fructose Corn Syrup or Corn Syrup. When you check out at the grocery store all those *delicious* snacks and sweets that you are surrounded by are filled with chemicals and fake ingredients. #uggg

Trust me, I know the struggle when

it comes to those cravings. I was once addicted to soda. I thought I couldn't live without it! Analyzing that soda is what started my journey. After merely googling the ingredients I discovered that it was unquestionably, not in the least bit healthy. I began to examine everything. I immediately quit drinking soda and eventually quit craving it. (Switching over to carbonated water helped with my carbonated craving.) At first I didn't necessarily enjoy it, but after time the sight of a soda made me queasy. #forreal

It definitely is hard at first learning all this about what we are consuming. I would go to the gas station for a beverage or snack and become incredibly depressed. I have now learned to just go where I *know* I have options. It makes it easier to just buy it in packs so I have a healthy option to bring with me when I'm out. It took me about 3 years to discover that they made ORGANIC soda. Oh MY! I was excited the day I found this! I now enjoy a soda every now and then

(I still prefer my sparkling water more), but when I do crave a soda I have a healthy option! #Dancing. The soda I found is made from spices and herbs. It sounds weird, but this is how it should be! The brand I choose is made with clove bud oil, cassia oil, cinnamon, nutmeg, caramel, vanilla extract, lemon, orange, lime extracts, and unbleached cane sugar. It does have 38 grams of sugar so I suggest sparingly, but if you must have a soda this is what I'd recommend. It tastes nearly the same and is WAY better for you! (Cheers to alternatives!) They also make soda sweetened with stevia. This is another great replacement for that soda with the HFCS. (6 packs in my area are about $3.00-$4.00. This is a better deal than grabbing a soda at a gas station everyday.) #JustSayin'

If you want to be healthier, but you have a deep hankering for soda and sweets, fear not! You don't have to give it up completely, go on a boring diet, or quit cold turkey and suffer with those withdraws. (If that's what you prefer, by all means- do it!) You just have to change your lifestyle a little bit. Find a local store that sells better options and then buy in bulk. Take your sweet treats with you and avoid that gas station trip. Finding alternatives is becoming easier and easier as time goes on. People are becoming more and more aware. The demand for natural and unprocessed foods is increasing. #exciting!

The candy or gummy bears I purchase for my daughters lunch (so she can be cool too) is made from fruit juice and unbleached cane sugar. There is chocolates made from pure ingredients as well. I also like making chocolate at home from raw, organic cacao (not to be mistaken for *cocoa*). There are a ton of easy and quick recipes online.

When I baked at home I *was* using just raw, organic, unrefined, herbally purified, fairly traded, sustainably produced, pesticide, and herbicide free cane sugar. (The white cane sugar you

usually see is very processed and **bleached**.)
There still isn't much, if any nutritional
value, but your body can process this a lot
easier than the majority of artificial
sweeteners. At least you're getting the
calories (15 calories per teaspoon) to go
with the sugar so your body is not "tricked."
You can also control the amount you use by
baking at home. There is also pure, organic,
raw honey as an option. There are a ton of
health benefits in honey a few being:
healthy weight management, natural
energy source, helps with allergies, etc. To
be honest I don't like the flavor that honey
adds to some baked goods or my coffee. I
definitely prefer that *real* sugar. (Honey
contains 15/20 calories per teaspoon.)
   So there you have it! That is how I
avoid all those artificial/chemical
sweeteners while I'm out and about and
still enjoy the luxury of continuously happy
taste buds. I personally stay away from
anything that is labeled "low-calorie" or
"sugar-free." It seems in the end there are

not any benefits to be reaped. I eat chocolate, candy, and drink occasional sodas. They are all naturally made and sweetened with either *unbleached cane sugar, cane sugar, or non-GMO organic stevia*. (Look on the back of the product's ingredient list.)

Unbleached cane sugar and non-GMO, organic stevia sugar in our sweet treats is unequivocally a healthier option. Moderation is the key. (Hopefully, we will soon see Luo Han Guo Fruit/Monk Fruit as the new sweetener of choice in our store bought products.)

Spending an extra dollar or two on a cleaner product is definitely worth it. If you are budgeting and it seems outrageous, just consider the potential future medical bills. From my own firsthand experience you will feel better, and have so much more energy!

Now, I completely understand that many people are looking for 0 calorie or low-calorie. Just the sight of 15-20 calories per teaspoon even makes ME cringe!

(Especially now that I'm nearing my 30's.) If you are looking for zero calories than the **Luo Han Guo Fruit (Monk Fruit)** _IS_ the answer. This sweetener seems to defy all odds.

Turn to the next page to discover the one and only...
The life-changing...
The impossible...
The answer to immortality...

Disclaimer: I am not God. I can not give immortality.

"The Immortal's Fruit"
(Ta-Ta-Ta-Dah!)

Psssh, who wants a taste of the sweetener from "The Immortals Fruit?" (ME! I DO. Count me in!)

I *must* go over **Luo Han Guo Fruit (Monk Fruit)** benefits one more time. This fruit is extraordinary! Let's review the pros again...

*0 calories per gram. (What!) This is the amazing part. This *naturally* has 0 calories.

In the beginning of this book I talked about "0 calories" or "low-calories" sabotaging your weight loss. So, how is this different? I will explain.

Monk fruit grows in the Asian regions. This fruit becomes rotten very quickly after it is harvested (this is the reason we don't see it in the U.S.). When it's *fresh,* it does technically contain carbohydrates and calories, but since it dies so quickly the trace amounts of fructose, glucose, and carbohydrates that it does contain is considered insignificant. If the fructose, glucose, and other components perish with the fruit- how is it sweet? Monk Fruit is not sweet from natural sugars like most fruits, but it is *very* sweet. (200-400 times sweeter than cane sugar.) Here is the exciting part! Here is why it doesn't sabotage your weight like artificial sweeteners do. It contains very powerful antioxidants called *mogrosides.* These antioxidants **metabolize differently** in the body. (Unlike natural or fake sugars.) Yes, it may be sweeter than cane sugar, but this amazing fruit contains no calories or carbs due to the miracle that the antioxidants are what give it its sweetness- not fructose, glucose, or any other naturally occurring sugar. This also allows for it to have hardly any effect on blood sugar which in turn may have a powerful **effect on diabetes**. Because of the 0 calories and 0 carbohydrates this also helps **prevent weight gain.** We can obtain the sweetness that we crave without the harmful side effects of table sugar, artificial sweeteners and GMOs found in most sweeteners. #WOW. #BlownAway

*0 Glycemic Index.** No high rush or crash later.

*The Benefits known in China for 800+ years.** (Come on U.S. of all the things we import from China- we didn't start with this!?)

*Good, clean taste.** I've had it- it taste just like cane sugar!

*Supports the immune system, digestive tract, glands, and respiratory system.** Monk Fruit has antimicrobial properties that keep proper bacterial balance. This in turn will assist with your immune system, the gut bacteria, helps fight diseases, disorders, and illnesses. It's all one full circle within your system! The antioxidants in the fruit also help prevent DNA damage as well! #livelonger #lookyounger

*May help with allergies. It calms the mast cells that release the chemicals such as histamine-which is associated with allergies and asthma.

*May help with Cancer. There have been countless studies proving that Monk Fruit has assisted in improving or eradicating cancer. The proteins in the fruit have powerful potent abilities to fight and reduce cancer. (Studies have shown that it has helped skin, breast and other cancers.)

*Fights Free Radicals. Oxidative stress plays a huge part in many diseases. This fruit is HIGH in antioxidants. Antioxidants have been known to reduce free radicals.

*Acts as an anti-inflammatory. Inflammation

can cause a lot of different problems in the body. Some of the medicine we use for inflammation can have harmful side effects. Monk Fruits has proven powerful anti-inflammatory properties.

*May decrease risk of heart disease. A study showed that this fruit prevented cholesterol from oxidizing. Which than, in turn, decreased plaque buildup in the arteries.

*Doesn't promote tooth decay. Monk Fruit has been proven to fight candida symptoms and oral thrush. It has natural antimicrobial agents to help fight infections.

*Considered one of the safest non-sugar sweeteners. (I'd say!)

*No known concerns. Currently there are no known side effects using this sweetener. (The use of this for 800+ years may be a good indication that this is safe…)

*Extracted naturally. The most common way that this sweetener is extracted is through water infusion. It is filtered and then dried to give you that sugary, grainy, powder extract.

Wow! Isn't this just music to your ears? I still can't believe this! From what I just read and researched Monk Fruits is *THE BEST* option for sweetening our food and beverages! Since writing this book I have switched over to this God-send deliciousness. It's perfect timing for me (I'm currently expecting my second baby.) This is truly an ideal alternative to help me keep my sweet intake on the low, low. Ya know? I'm always hungry, I love to bake, and I love a little sweet in my coffee. #yay *(Currently doing a dance!) It is becoming more popular so maybe soon we will have this in our candy bars instead of unbleached cane sugar for our healthy choices!

When purchasing this you still have to read the little ingredient list on the back. There are brands that mix it with dextrose and other artificial ingredients. So just keep a lookout! The one I currently have is a pure Monk Fruit extract by Smart138. I purchase it online**.** There is a popular brand that is mixed with **erythritol**. From my research, as long as you use organic and non-GMO erythritol it should be safe, but pure, plain, and simple Monk Fruit is always the best option.

Monk Fruit can still be difficult to find in stores, but if you google it you will find it for around $5.00-$10.00 online. There definitely is wholesome, undiluted, and clean brands. Isn't this exciting! Nature gave us 0 calories! We don't need chemicals or labs to offer us a better lifestyle- nature has come through once again. Is this not the best thing you've ever read or maybe the best piece of information you've learned today?

Contemplation

Until I began my little journey on researching W.T.H. is in our food I didn't even realize what I was feeding my own self and family. We, as Americans, are so accustomed to **warning** labels nowadays. It's "normal" and we ignore it. We overlook things like this for various reasons; such as: our parents ate it, a favorite lifelong snack, or it says "no-calories," etc. Similar to the warning labels on cigarettes and alcohol. It gives us a short *fix* to feel good at the time, but the consequences are far more dangerous than the small reward. Is it possible our food is made differently than when the product first came out in the 40's, 50's, or 60's? Do we, by chance use different preservatives and sweeteners than we did originally? It's important to take all this into consideration.

After reading the potential side effects of artificial sweeteners, will you still let your children get a pack of gum while you're standing in line at the grocery store? Surely do as you wish, just think about the cons of artificial sweeteners before you give them to your children or friends. One dose of course, will not hurt, but over a period of time it can definitely cause harm. Let us start treating our families to healthier alternatives. It takes a small bit of work, like reading a label, or maybe began shopping at your local health food store. Please don't be fooled by flashy packaging that is meant to attract our kids. We together can take responsibility for the health and wellness of our friends, family, and ourselves causing the world of artificial to disappear one purchase at a time.

 Fun Fact: (or sad fact. lol) Did you know that just 200 years ago the average American ate about 2 pounds of sugar a year. Now the average American eats about 152 pounds of sugar every year. That is roughly 3 pounds of sugar a week! WOAH! MMM… Maybe we should invest in some of that Monk Fruit? What do you think?

Welp, I really hope you enjoyed this little read and gained a little insight.

Just please remember to research all of it yourself before you finalize your own opinion. I had fun writing and researching. Remember: **YOUR HEALTH DOES MATTER**! **YOU MATTER!** Let's make a change one ingredient at a time..

For nourishing recipes, cool lifestyle ideas, and fun researched information follow me
@victoriapetraz

NOTES:

NOTES:

References

www.polyols.org
www.sweetenerbook.com
www.health.com
www.naturalhealth365.com
www.sugar-sweet-sweetener-guide.com\
www.naturalhealth365.com
www.foodnavigator-usa.com
www.cyclamat.org
www.nlm.nih.gov
www.snopes.com
www.m.cancer.org
www.articles.mercola.com
www.diethealthclub.com
www.liveto110.comcomplete-list-of-artifici
al-sweeteners/
www.aspartame.org/about/benefits
www.fda.gov/food/ingredientspackaginglab
eling/foodadditivesingredients/ucm397725.
htm
www.authoritynutrition.com
www.goldenrule.com/health-wellness/the-
pros-and-cons-of-artificial-sweeteners/

www.mercola.com/sites/articles/archives/2009/artificial-sweeteners-more-dangerous-than-you-ever-imagined.aspx

www.mercola/sites/archives/2014/12/23/artificial-sweeteners-confuse-body.aspx

www.nutritionexpress.com/article+index/vitamins+supplements+2/showarticle.aspx?101=120

www.osha.gov.publications/osha3144.html

www.realdiabetestruth.com/advantame-aspartame-artificial-sweetener

www.fitnessfortravel.com/is-maltodextrin-bad-for-you/

www.sweetpoison.com/aspartame-side-effects.html

www.en.wikipedia.org/wiki

www.cyclamate.org

www.mobile.foodnavigator-usa.com/regulations/steviol/natural-says-new-class-action-lawsuit

www.nhs.uk

www.sugar-sweetener-guide.com/cyclamate.html

www.wisegeek.com/what-is-isomalt.htm

www.blog.amberlynchocolates.com/maltito
l-beauty-or-beast
www.theingredientdatabase.wordpress.co
m/2012/05/20/neohesperidin-dihydrochalc
one/
www.codexalimentarius.net/gsfaoline/addi
tives/details.html?id=340
www.codexalimentarius.net/asfaonline/add
itives/details.html?id=104
www.medicinenet.com/artificial_sweetener
s/page10.html
www.livestrong.com/article/414517-what-i
s-acesulfame-potassium/
www.foodmaters.tv
www.thrivemarket.com
www.iquitsugar.com
www.karma-free-cooking.com
https:/dhhs.nh.gov/dphs/nhp/documents/sugar
.pdf
www.howfoodgrows.com
www.iherb.com
www.golbalhealingcenter.com
www.articles.mercola.com
www.drhyman.com

www.emedicinehealth.com
www.health.com
www.sugar.org
www.befoodsmart.com
www.youtube.com/watch?v=s-4RR7XDyHs
www.naturalhealth365.com/monk-fruit.html/
https://www.draxe.com/monk

Made in the USA
Middletown, DE
03 December 2022

16773010R00066